REVITALIZE 2024

A Comprehensive Juicing Guide to Health and Wellness

Meredith .A. Greene

Table of Contents

Introduction

Welcome to Juicing! Embark on a journey towards better health and vitality through juicing. Discover the essence of juicing, its benefits, and how this book will serve as your guide to integrating this powerful health practice into your daily life. Juicing is the process of extracting juice from fresh fruits and vegetables, creating nutrient-rich beverages that are easy to digest and quick to absorb. This practice involves separating the liquid from the pulp, resulting in a drink packed with vitamins, minerals, and antioxidants. By consuming juices, you can significantly increase your intake of essential nutrients, promoting overall health and wellness. This book is designed to be your comprehensive guide to the world of juicing. You will learn about the different types of juicers, the best produce to use, and the nutritional benefits of various fruits and vegetables. I will provide practical tips on selecting and storing your ingredients, maintaining your juicer, and creating delicious and balanced juice recipes. You will find a variety of recipes tailored to different health goals, from energy-boosting morning blends to calming evening concoctions. Additionally, the book offers structures juicing programs for detoxification, weight loss, and specific health conditions, helping you to achieve your wellness objectives through targeted juicing strategies. By integrating the knowledge and practices outlined in this book, you will be well-equipped to harness the full potential of juicing, leading you towards a healthier, more vibrant life.

Welcome To The World Of Juicing!

What is Juicing? Juicing extracts the liquid from fresh fruits and vegetables, preserving essential vitamins, minerals, and phytonutrients. This process allows you to consume a concentrated amount of nutrients in a convenient, delicious form.

Benefits of Juicing; Learn how juicing can boost your nutrient intake, support detoxification, improve digestion, and enhance your overall energy levels. Explore the diverse benefits that make juicing an excellent addition to a healthy lifestyle. Juicing offers a convenient way to consume a variety of fruits and vegetables, ensuring you get a broad spectrum of essential vitamins and minerals. By extracting the juice, you retain the most concentrated form of nutrients, which can lead to improved health outcomes. Juicing allows you to easily incorporate a wider range of produce into your diet, including those you might not typically eat whole. One of the key benefits of juicing is its ability to support detoxification. The abundance of antioxidants in fresh juices helps to neutralize harmful free radicals and cleanse the body of toxins. This can promote better liver function and enhance your body's natural detox processes. Regular juicing can lead to clearer skin, improved mental clarity, and increased vitality. Improved digestion is another significant benefit of juicing. Without the fiber, your digestive system can absorb nutrients more quickly and efficiently. This is particularly beneficial for individuals with digestive issues, as it allows their bodies to obtain the necessary nutrients without the additional burden of breaking down fibrous foods. Juicing can also promote a healthy gut flora, which is essential for overall digestive health. Juicing is also known for its ability to boost energy levels. The quick absorption of nutrients provides an immediate source of energy, making it an excellent option for a morning pick-me-up or a pre-workout boost. Unlike caffeinated beverages, juices provide sustained energy without the crash, thanks to their natural sugars and balanced nutrient profile. Furthermore, juicing can aid in weight management. By replacing high-calorie, low-nutrient foods with nutrient-dense juices, you can reduce your overall calorie intake while still feeling satisfied and nourished. Juicing can help curb cravings and reduce the likelihood of overeating, making it a valuable tool in a balanced weight loss plan. Finally, regular juicing can strengthen your immune system. The high concentration of vitamins, particularly vitamin C, and other immune-boosting nutrients found in fresh juices can help your body fend off infections and illnesses. Incorporating a variety of fruits and vegetables into your juices ensures that you are getting a comprehensive array of nutrients to support overall health and resilience. Juicing is a powerful practice that can significantly enhance your nutrient intake, support detoxification, improve digestion, boost energy levels, aid in weight management, and strengthen your immune system. By making juicing a regular part of your routine, you can experience these diverse benefits and enjoy a healthier, more vibrant lifestyle.

How to Use This Book

This guide is designed to be both informative and practical. Whether you read it cover to cover or jump to sections of interest, you'll find actionable tips and recipes to incorporate juicing into your routine effectively. So enjoy!

Chapter 1: The Basics of Juicing

What I need To Get Started

Essentials Equipment

Getting started with juicing requires a few essential pieces of equipment to ensure you have everything you need for a smooth and enjoyable experience. First and foremost, you'll need a good quality juicer. Additionally, you'll want a sharp knife for cutting produce, a cutting board, and a peeler for certain fruits and vegetables. A fine mesh strainer or nut milk bag can be useful for straining pulp if you prefer a smoother juice. To store your juice, invest in some airtight glass containers. Lastly, a brush for cleaning your juicer□s parts will help maintain hygiene and longevity of your equipment.

Choosing the Right Juicer

Choosing the right juicer is crucial for achieving the best results based on your needs and budget. There are three main types of juicers: centrifugal juicers, masticating (slow) juicers, and manual juicers. Each type has its own advantages and price points.

Types of Juicers: Affordable Options

#Centrifugal Juicers

Centrifugal juicers are the most common and typically the most affordable option. They use a fast-spinning blade to chop up the produce and then spin it at high speed to separate the juice from the pulp. These juicers are great for beginners due to their speed and ease of use. However, they can be noisy and may not extract as much juice from leafy greens as other types. Prices for centrifugal juicers range from $50 to $150. Some popular models in this category include the Hamilton Beach Juicer Machine ($60) and the Breville Juice Fountain Compact ($100).

Masticating (Slow) Juicers

Masticating juicers, also known as slow or cold-press juicers, use an auger to crush and press the produce, extracting juice more slowly but more efficiently. They are excellent for retaining nutrients and extracting juice from leafy greens and wheatgrass. While they are generally more expensive than centrifugal juicers, they provide higher juice yields and quieter operation. Prices for masticating juicers typically range from $150 to $400. Notable models include the Omega J8006HDS Nutrition Center Juicer ($300) and the Aico Slow Masticating Juicer ($150).

Manual Juicers

Manual juicers are the most budget-friendly and portable option, ideal for those who juice occasionally or prefer a hands-on approach. These juicers operate by using a hand-crank mechanism to press and squeeze juice from the produce. They are especially effective for juicing citrus fruits but can also handle other fruits and vegetables with a bit more effort. Manual juicers are quiet, easy to clean, and very affordable, with prices typically ranging from $20 to $80. Popular choices include the Zulay Professional Citrus Juicer ($50) and the Lexen GP27 Manual Wheatgrass Juicer ($60).

When choosing a juicer, consider what types of produce you plan to juice most frequently, your budget, and how much time you're willing to spend on preparation and cleaning. This will help you find the best juicer to meet your needs and ensure a satisfying juicing experience.

Understanding Ingredients

Fruits

Fruits are the foundation of many juice recipes, offering natural sweetness, vibrant colors, and a wealth of nutrients. Common fruits used in juicing include apples, oranges, berries, and citrus fruits, each contributing unique flavors and health benefits. Apples, for instance, add a sweet base, while citrus fruits like oranges and lemons provide a zesty tang. Berries are packed with antioxidants, and exotic fruits like mangoes and pineapples bring tropical notes to your juice blends. Understanding the properties of different fruits can help you create balanced and delicious juice combinations.

Vegetables

Vegetables are an excellent addition to juices, bringing a range of flavors and nutritional benefits. Leafy greens like spinach and kale are popular for their high vitamin and mineral content, while cucumbers and celery add a refreshing, hydrating element. Root vegetables such as carrots and beets offer earthy sweetness and vibrant color.

Including a variety of vegetables in your juice not only enhances its health benefits but also helps to balance the sweetness of the fruits, creating a more complex and satisfying flavor profile.

Herbs and Spices

Herbs and spices can elevate your juices by adding depth and complexity to the flavors. Fresh herbs like mint, basil, and parsley bring a burst of freshness and can complement both fruit and vegetable juices. Spices such as ginger, turmeric, and cinnamon offer a warm, aromatic touch and have numerous health benefits, including anti-inflammatory properties. Experimenting with different herbs and spices can help you discover new flavor combinations and boost the overall nutritional value of your juices.

Preparation and Storage

Washing and Preparing Produce

Properly washing and preparing your produce is crucial for both the quality and safety of your juices. Start by thoroughly rinsing fruits and vegetables under cold water to remove dirt, pesticides, and any other contaminants. For produce with thick skins or rinds, such as cucumbers and oranges, consider peeling them before juicing. Cut larger fruits and vegetables into smaller pieces that will fit easily into your juicer. Removing seeds and pits is also important to prevent any bitterness and to protect your juicer from damage. Taking the time to properly prepare your produce ensures that your juice is clean, safe, and delicious.

Storing Juices for Freshness

To maintain the freshness and nutritional value of your juices, proper storage is essential. Freshly made juice should ideally be consumed immediately, but if you need to store it, use an airtight container to minimize exposure to air and prevent oxidation. Glass containers are preferable as they do not retain odors or flavors and are easy to clean. Store your juice in the refrigerator and consume it within 24 to 48 hours for the best taste and nutrient retention. If you want to keep juice for a longer period, consider freezing it in individual portions, which can be thawed as needed. By following these storage tips, you can enjoy fresh, healthy juice anytime.

Chapter 2: Juicing for Health

Juicing for Detoxification

Detoxification through juicing is a popular method to cleanse the body, enhance energy levels, and improve overall health. This chapter delves into the principles of juicing for detoxification, provides recipes, and offers guidance on how to maximize the benefits of a juice cleanse.

Understanding Detoxification

Detoxification is the process of removing toxins from the body. Our bodies are naturally equipped with organs like the liver, kidneys, and lymphatic system to detoxify and eliminate waste. However, modern lifestyles, with their exposure to pollutants, processed foods, and stress, can overload these systems. Juicing can provide a concentrated source of nutrients that support the body□s natural detoxification processes.

Benefits of Juicing for Detoxification

Nutrient-Rich: Fresh juices are packed with vitamins, minerals, and antioxidants that aid in the detoxification process.

Hydration: Juicing increases your fluid intake, which helps flush out toxins. Alkalizing: Many fruits and vegetables are alkaline, which can help balance the body□spH and reduce acidity.

Improved Digestion: Juices are easy to digest and can give the digestive system a break from processing solid foods.

Increased Energy: Many people report higher energy levels and mental clarity during and after a juice cleanse.

Key Ingredients for Detox Juices

Leafy Greens: Spinach, kale, and parsley are rich in chlorophyll, which helps cleanse the blood.

Citrus Fruits: Lemons, limes, and grapefruits are high in vitamin C and aid in liver detoxification.

Root Vegetables: Beets and carrots are excellent for liver health and help in the elimination of toxins.

Cucumbers: High in water content, they aid in hydration and flush out toxins. Ginger and Turmeric: These roots have anti-inflammatory properties and support liver function.

When preparing for a Juice Cleanse

It's not advisable to just start like that without doing these things first:

Consult a Healthcare Professional: Before starting a juice cleanse, especially if you have any medical conditions, consult with a healthcare provider.

Plan Your Cleanse: Decide on the duration of your cleanse. Beginners might start with a 1-3 day cleanse, while more experienced individuals might opt for 5-7 days.

Ease In and Out: Gradually ease into the cleanse by reducing processed foods, caffeine, and alcohol a few days before starting. Similarly, ease out of the cleanse by slowly reintroducing solid foods.

Sample Juice Cleanse Plan

Day 1: Preparation

Morning: Warm water with lemon

Breakfast: Green Juice (spinach, cucumber, apple, lemon, ginger)

Mid-Morning: Herbal tea

Lunch: Carrot and Beet Juice (carrot, beet, apple, ginger)

Afternoon

Snack: Coconut water

Dinner: Citrus Juice (grapefruit, orange, lemon, turmeric)

Evening: Herbal tea

Day 2-3: Cleanse

Morning: Warm water with lemon

Breakfast: Green Juice

Mid-Morning: Herbal tea or detox tea

Lunch: Beet and Carrot Juice

Afternoon Snack: Green Juice

Dinner: Citrus Juice

Evening: Herbal tea or detox tea

Day 4: Post-Cleanse

Morning: Warm water with lemon

Breakfast: Smoothie (banana, spinach, almond milk)

Mid-Morning: Fresh fruit or light snack

Lunch: Light vegetable soup or salad

Afternoon Snack: Fresh fruit

Dinner: Steamed vegetables with a small portion of protein (like fish or tofu)

Evening: Herbal tea

Tips for a Successful Juice Cleanse

Stay Hydrated: Drink plenty of water and herbal teas throughout the day to stay hydrated and help flush out toxins.

Listen to Your Body: If you feel dizzy or excessively tired, consider having a light snack like a handful of nuts or a piece of fruit.

Rest: Allow your body to rest and avoid strenuous activities during the cleanse.

Support Digestion: Gentle yoga, deep breathing exercises, and dry brushing can help support the detoxification process.

Post-Cleanse: Maintaining Benefits

Reintroduce Foods Gradually: Start with light, easily digestible foods like fruits, vegetables, and smoothies.

Maintain a Balanced Diet: Incorporate a variety of whole foods, including lean proteins, healthy fats, and complex carbohydrates.

Continue Juicing: Incorporate fresh juices into your daily or weekly routine to continue receiving their nutritional benefits. Explore the science and benefits of detoxifying your body through juicing. Find recipes specifically designed to help cleanse and rejuvenate your system.

Why Detoxify?

Detoxification is an essential process for maintaining optimal health and well-being. Here are several reasons why detoxifying through juicing can be beneficial:

1. Elimination of Toxins

Our bodies are constantly exposed to toxins from various sources, including processed foods, environmental pollutants, chemicals, and even stress. Over time, these toxins can accumulate and hinder the body's natural functions. Detoxifying helps to:

Reduce Toxin Load: By eliminating harmful substances, you can reduce the burden on your liver, kidneys, and other detoxification organs.

1. Improve Organ Function: Supporting the body's natural detox pathways can enhance the efficiency of the liver, kidneys, and lymphatic system.

2. Enhanced Nutrient Absorption: Detoxifying through juicing can improve the body's ability to absorb essential nutrients. Freshly made juices are rich in vitamins,

minerals, and enzymes that are easily absorbed by the body, providing a quick and potent nutrient boost. Boosted Immune System: A nutrient-rich diet helps strengthen the immune system, making the body more resilient to infections and diseases.

Increased Energy Levels: Enhanced nutrient absorption can lead to higher energy levels and reduced fatigue.

3. It improves Digestion: A juice cleanse can give your digestive system a break from processing solid foods, allowing it to reset and rejuvenate.

Gut Health: Juicing provides a source of easily digestible nutrients that can help soothe and heal the digestive tract.

Reduced Bloating: Many people experience reduced bloating and improved bowel movements during and after a juice cleanse.

4. Weight Management: Juicing can be an effective tool for weight management. While it is not a long-term weight loss solution, it can kickstart healthier eating habits and help break cycles of poor dietary choices.

5. Calorie Control: Juicing can help you control calorie intake while still providing essential nutrients.

Craving Reduction: A cleanse can help reset taste buds and reduce cravings for unhealthy foods.

6. Mental Clarity and Emotional Well-Being: Detoxifying can have positive effects on mental clarity and emotional well-being. Many people report feeling more focused,

clear-headed, and emotionally balanced during and after a cleanse.

7.Reduced Stress: Eliminating toxins can help reduce the physical and mental stress on the body.

Improved Mood: Nutrient-dense juices can support neurotransmitter production, leading to improved mood and mental clarity.

8. For a clearer Skin: The skin is a major organ of detoxification, and cleansing can help improve its appearance. By removing toxins from the body, you may notice several positive changes in your skin, such as:

Improved Hydration: Your skin might appear more hydrated and plump due to the increased intake of water and nutrients from the juice.

Enhanced Glow: The vitamins and antioxidants in the juice, like Vitamin C and E, can give your skin a natural glow and brightness.

Reduced Acne: Juices rich in anti-inflammatory ingredients and low in sugar can help reduce acne and blemishes.

Even Skin Tone: Regular intake of healthy juices may help in reducing hyperpigmentation and dark spots, leading to a more even skin tone.

Softness and Smoothness: The nutrients in juices can improve the texture of your skin, making it feel softer and smoother.

Fewer Wrinkles: Antioxidants in juices can help combat free radicals, potentially slowing down the aging process and reducing the appearance of fine lines and wrinkles.

Reduction in Acne and Blemishes: Clearer skin and reduced inflammation. Improved Skin Tone and Texture: Healthier, more radiant skin.

Here are some home made juice recipes that are great for skin care:

Radiant Glow Juice

This juice is packed with Vitamin C and antioxidants to brighten your complexion and give your skin a natural glow.

Ingredients:

2 oranges (peeled)

1 carrot

1/2 cucumber

1/2 lemon (peeled)

1/2 inch piece of ginger

1/4 teaspoon turmeric powder (optional)

Instructions:

Wash all the ingredients thoroughly.

Peel the oranges, lemon, and ginger.

Cut the carrot, cucumber, and ginger into pieces that fit your juicer.

Juice all the ingredients together.

Stir in turmeric powder if desired and enjoy!

Green Goddess Juice

This juice is rich in vitamins A, C, and E, which are essential for healthy skin. It's also incredibly hydrating.

Ingredients:

1 cucumber

1 handful of spinach

1 handful of kale

1 green apple (optional for sweetness)

1/2 lemon (peeled)

1/2 inch piece of ginger

Instructions:

Wash all the ingredients.

Peel the lemon and ginger.

Cut the cucumber, apple, and ginger into pieces that fit your juicer.

Juice all the ingredients, starting with the leafy greens.

Stir and drink immediately.

Berry Beauty Juice

This juice is loaded with antioxidants from the berries, which help combat free radicals and support collagen production.

Ingredients:

1 cup of strawberries

1/2 cup of blueberries

1/2 cup of raspberries

1 apple (optional for sweetness)

1/2 cucumber

1/2 lemon (peeled)

Instructions:

Wash all the ingredients thoroughly.

Peel the lemon.

Cut the apple and cucumber into pieces that fit your juicer.

Juice all the ingredients together.

Stir and enjoy!

Aloe & Pineapple Skin Soother

This juice is perfect for soothing and healing your skin from the inside out, thanks to the aloe vera and pineapple.

Ingredients:

1/2 cup fresh aloe vera gel (from an aloe leaf)

1 cup pineapple chunks

1/2 cucumber

1/2 lemon (peeled)

1/4 cup coconut water (optional for added hydration)

Instructions:

Wash all the ingredients.

Cut the pineapple, cucumber, and lemon into pieces that fit your juicer.

Scoop out the fresh aloe vera gel from the leaf.

Juice everything together, including the aloe gel.Add coconut water if desired, stir, and enjoy!

9. It prevents Chronic Diseases

Long-term exposure to toxins and poor dietary habits can contribute to the development of chronic diseases. Regular detoxification can help reduce the risk of conditions such as:

Heart Disease: By improving cardiovascular health through a nutrient-rich diet.

Diabetes: By promoting balanced blood sugar levels.

Inflammatory Conditions: By reducing overall inflammation in the body.

8. Alkalizing the Body.

Many fruits and vegetables used in juicing are alkaline, which can help balance the body's pH levels. An alkaline diet is believed to:

Reduce Acidity: Lower the risk of chronic diseases associated with high acidity. Promote Overall Health: Support various bodily functions and improve overall health.

Detox Juices Recipe:

 Green Detox Juice

Ingredients:1 cucumber

2 celery stalks

1 cup spinach

1 apple

1 lemon, peeled

1-inch piece of ginger

Instructions: Wash all ingredients thoroughly. Chop produce into juicer-friendly sizes. Juice all ingredients and stir well. Serve immediately or store in an airtight container for up to 24 hours.

Boosting Immunity with Juices

Identify key ingredients that enhance your immune system and discover immunity-boosting juice recipes to keep you healthy and resilient.

Immunity-Boosting Juice Recipe: Citrus Ginger Zinger

Ingredients:2 oranges, peeled

1 lemon, peeled

1 carrot

1-inch piece of ginger

Instructions: Wash all ingredients.

Peel citrus fruits and ginger.

Juice all ingredients and mix well.

Consume immediately for best results.

Juicing for Weight Loss

Understand how juicing can support your weight loss goals by providing nutrient-dense, low-calorie options. Access a variety of weight loss juice recipes to aid your journey.

Weight Loss Juice Recipe: Cucumber Melon Slimmer

Ingredients:1 cucumber

1/2 honeydew melon

1 green apple

1 handful of mint leaves

Instructions: Wash and chop all ingredients.

Juice all ingredients together.

Stir well and enjoy immediately.

Energy and Vitality: Learn about energizing ingredients that can naturally boost your vitality. Find recipes tailored to give you a quick and sustained energy lift.

Energy-Boosting Recipe: Morning Energy Blast

Ingredients:

2 apples

1 orange, peeled

1 beet1-inch piece of ginger

Instructions:

Wash and chop all ingredients.

Juice all ingredients and mix well.

Drink immediately for a burst of energy.

Juicing for Weight Loss

How Juicing Can Help?

Juicing can be an effective tool for weight loss when used as part of a balanced diet and healthy lifestyle.

 Here's how juicing can assist in shedding those extra pounds: Low-calorie, Nutrient-Dense Option: Juices made from fresh fruits and vegetables are typically low in calories but rich in essential nutrients, vitamins, and minerals. This means you can consume fewer calories without sacrificing nutritional intake.

Promotes Satiety: Certain fruits and vegetables contain high amounts of fiber, which helps you feel full longer. Although juicing removes some fiber, including pulp in your juice or complementing your juice with fiber-rich foods can help maintain satiety.

Reduces Cravings: Fresh juices can help reduce cravings for unhealthy snacks and sweets. When your body receives the nutrients it needs, it□s less likely to crave junk food. Increases Vegetable Intake: Many people find it challenging to eat the recommended servings of vegetables each day. Juicing makes it easier to consume a variety of vegetables, ensuring you get a broad spectrum of nutrients that support weight loss and overall health.

Boosts Metabolism: Certain ingredients, like ginger and lemon, can help boost your metabolism, making it easier for your body to burn calories more efficiently.

Detoxifies the Body: A juice cleanse can help remove toxins from the body, which can improve digestion, reduce bloating, and enhance overall bodily functions. A cleaner, more efficient system can support weight loss efforts.

Weight Loss Juice Recipes

Green Fat Burner Juice

Ingredients: Spinach, kale, green apple, cucumber, lemon, ginger.

Benefits: Packed with leafy greens that provide essential vitamins and minerals while keeping calories low. The lemon and ginger help boost metabolism.

Carrot and Apple Detox Juice

Ingredients: Carrots, green apples, celery, lemon.

Benefits: High in fiber and low in calories, this juice supports digestion and detoxification.

Citrus Slimming Juice

Ingredients: Grapefruit, orange, lemon, turmeric. Benefits: Citrus fruits are low in calories and high in vitamin C, which aids in fat metabolism.

Beet and Berry Metabolism Booster

Ingredients: Beets, blueberries, strawberries, ginger.

Benefits: Beets and berries are rich in antioxidants and nutrients that support metabolic health and energy production.

Energy and Vitality

To maintain high energy levels and vitality, it's crucial to incorporate ingredients into your juices that naturally boost energy.

Energizing Ingredients:

Here are some top energizing ingredients:

Spinach: Rich in iron and nitrates, spinach helps improve oxygen transport in the blood, which can boost energy levels and endurance. Beets: Beets are high in natural nitrates, which can enhance blood flow and improve athletic performance and stamina.

Ginger: Known for its anti-inflammatory properties, ginger can improve circulation and reduce fatigue, making it an excellent addition to energy-boosting juices. Citrus Fruits: Oranges, lemons, and grapefruits are high in vitamin C and antioxidants, which help reduce fatigue and increase energy levels.

Apples: Apples are a good source of natural sugars and fiber, providing a quick energy boost while helping to stabilize blood sugar levels.

Carrots: High in beta-carotene and antioxidants, carrots support overall health and can help improve energy levels. Celery: Celery is hydrating and contains natural salts and minerals that help replenish the body and support sustained energy.

Berries: Blueberries, strawberries, and raspberries are packed with antioxidants and vitamins that help fight fatigue and improve mental clarity.

Energy-Boosting Juice Recipes

Green Energy Juice

Ingredients: Spinach, cucumber, green apple, celery, lemon, ginger. Benefits: A powerful blend of greens and ginger to boost energy, support digestion, and hydrate the body. Citrus Energizer Juice

Ingredients: Oranges, grapefruit, lemon, turmeric.

Benefits: This juice is packed with vitamin C and antioxidants that help reduce fatigue and boost the immune system.

Berry Blast Juice

Ingredients: Blueberries, strawberries, raspberries, apple, spinach. Benefits: Berries and spinach provide a rich source of antioxidants and vitamins that enhance mental clarity and energy levels.

Beetroot Power Juice

Ingredients: Beets, carrots, apple, ginger.

Benefits: This combination supports blood flow, improves oxygen transport, and provides a steady source of natural energy.

Chapter 3: Specific Health Concerns

Juices for Digestive Health

Benefits for Digestion

Proper digestion is crucial for overall health and well-being. Juices that aid digestion typically contain ingredients high in fiber, enzymes, and other nutrients that help to maintain a healthy digestive system. These juices can help with issues such as constipation, bloating, and indigestion.

~ Digestive Health Juice Recipes

1. Ginger Carrot Juice

   - Ingredients:

     - 4 carrots

     - 1 apple

     - 1-inch piece of ginger

     - 1 lemon (juiced)

   - Instructions:

     1. Wash all the ingredients thoroughly.

     2. Cut the carrots and apple into pieces that will fit into your juicer.

     3. Peel the ginger.

     4. Run the carrots, apple, and ginger through the juicer.

     5. Stir in the lemon juice.

6. Serve immediately.

2. Aloe Vera Pineapple Juice

- Ingredients:

    - 1 cup fresh pineapple chunks

    - 1 cucumber

    - 2 tablespoons aloe vera gel (freshly extracted)

    - 1 lemon (juiced)

- Instructions:

    1. Wash and peel the cucumber, then cut it into chunks.

    2. Combine the pineapple, cucumber, and aloe vera gel in a blender.

    3. Blend until smooth.

    4. Strain the juice if desired.

    5. Stir in the lemon juice and serve.

Heart Health Juices

Ingredients for a Healthy Heart

Heart-healthy juices often include ingredients rich in antioxidants, vitamins, and minerals that support cardiovascular health. These ingredients help to lower blood pressure, reduce cholesterol levels, and improve overall heart function.

Heart-Healthy Juice Recipes

1. Beetroot Berry Juice

   - Ingredients:

      - 2 beetroots

      - 1 cup strawberries

      - 1 orange

      - 1-inch piece of ginger

   - Instructions:

      1. Wash all the ingredients thoroughly.

      2. Peel the beetroots and ginger.

      3. Cut the beetroots, strawberries, and orange into pieces.

      4. Run all ingredients through the juicer.

      5. Stir well and serve.

2. Spinach Apple Juice

   - Ingredients:

- 2 cups spinach

- 2 apples

- 1 cucumber

- 1 lemon (juiced)

-Instructions:

1. Wash all the ingredients thoroughly.

2. Core the apples and cut them into pieces.

3. Peel the cucumber if desired, and cut into chunks.

4. Run the spinach, apples, and cucumber through the juicer.

5. Stir in the lemon juice and serve.

Juicing for Skin Health

Nutrients for Glowing Skin

Skin-enhancing juices typically contain ingredients rich in vitamins A, C, and E, as well as antioxidants and other nutrients that promote healthy, glowing skin. These juices help to hydrate the skin, improve elasticity, and reduce signs of aging.

Skin-Enhancing Juice Recipes

1. Cucumber Mint Juice

- Ingredients:

    - 2 cucumbers

    - 1 green apple

    - 1 handful of fresh mint leaves

    - 1 lemon (juiced)

- Instructions:

    1. Wash all the ingredients thoroughly.

    2. Peel the cucumbers if desired, and cut into chunks.

    3. Core the apple and cut into pieces.

    4. Run the cucumbers, apple, and mint leaves through the juicer.

    5. Stir in the lemon juice and serve.

2. Carrot Orange Juice

- Ingredients:

    - 4 carrots

    - 2 oranges

    - 1-inch piece of turmeric root

    - 1-inch piece of ginger

- Instructions:

1. Wash all the ingredients thoroughly.

2. Peel the carrots, oranges, turmeric, and ginger.

3. Cut the ingredients into pieces that will fit into your juicer.

4. Run all ingredients through the juicer.

5. Stir well and serve.

3. Carrot Glow

Ingredients:

4 carrots

1 apple

1 orange, peeled

1-inch piece of turmeric root

Instructions:

Wash and chop all ingredients.

Juice all ingredients and stir well.

Drink immediately for best results.

Managing Blood Sugar with Juices

Low Glycemic Index Ingredients

Juices that help manage blood sugar levels typically include low glycemic index ingredients, which help to avoid spikes in blood sugar. These ingredients help to maintain stable energy levels and overall health.

Blood Sugar Balance Juice Recipes

1. Green Apple Celery Juice

   - Ingredients:

     - 2 green apples

     - 4 celery stalks

     - 1 cucumber

     - 1 lemon (juiced)

   -Instructions:

     1. Wash all the ingredients thoroughly.

     2. Core the apples and cut them into pieces.

     3. Cut the celery and cucumber into chunks.

     4. Run the apples, celery, and cucumber through the juicer.

     5. Stir in the lemon juice and serve.

2. Berry Spinach Juice

   - Ingredients:

      - 1 cup mixed berries (strawberries, blueberries, raspberries)

      - 2 cups spinach

      - 1 green apple

      - 1 lemon (juiced)

   - Instructions:

      1. Wash all the ingredients thoroughly.

      2. Core the apple and cut it into pieces.

      3. Run the berries, spinach, and apple through the juicer.

      4. Stir in the lemon juice and serve.

~ Juices for Anti-Inflammation

Anti-Inflammatory Ingredients

Juices that help reduce inflammation typically contain ingredients rich in antioxidants and anti-inflammatory compounds such as ginger, turmeric, and leafy greens. These ingredients can help to reduce inflammation throughout the body and improve overall health.

Anti-Inflammatory Juice Recipes

Turmeric Ginger Juice

Ingredients:

4 carrots

2 apples

1-inch piece of turmeric root

1-inch piece of ginger

1 lemon (juiced)

-Instructions:

1.Wash all the ingredients thoroughly.

2. Peel the carrots, apples, turmeric, and ginger.

3.Cut the ingredients into pieces that will fit into your juicer.

4. Run all ingredients through the juicer.

5.Stir in the lemon juice and serve.

Pineapple Cucumber Juice

Ingredients:

1 cup pineapple chunks

1 cucumber1-inch piece of ginger

1 handful of spinach

Instructions:

1. Wash all the ingredients thoroughly.

2. Peel the cucumber and ginger.

3.Cut the cucumber, pineapple, and ginger into chunks.

4. Run all ingredients through the juicer.

5.Stir well and serve.

Diabetic-Friendly Juices

Juices that are suitable for diabetics typically include ingredients with a low glycemic index to avoid spikes in blood sugar. These juices can help to maintain stable blood sugar levels and provide essential nutrients.

Diabetic-Friendly Juice Recipes

Green Veggie Juice

- Ingredients:

2 cups spinach

1 cucumber

1 green apple

1 lemon (juiced)

- Instructions:

1. Wash all the ingredients thoroughly.

2. Peel the cucumber if desired, and cut into chunks.

3. Core the apple and cut into pieces.

4. Run the spinach, cucumber, and apple through the juicer.

5. Stir in the lemon juice and serve.

Berry Citrus Juice

-Ingredients:

1 cup mixed berries (strawberries, blueberries, raspberries)

1 orange

1 lemon (juiced)

1 handful of kale

-Instructions:

1.Wash all the ingredients thoroughly.

2.Peel the orange.

3. Run the berries, orange, and kale through the juicer.

4. Stir in the lemon juice and serve.

THIS BLANK SPACE IS INTENTIONAL AND HAS BEEN DELIBERATELY INCLUDED TO ENHANCE THE READING EXPERIENCE. PLEASE CONTINUE WITH THE NEXT PAGE.

Chapter 4: Juicing for Fitness

Pre-Workout Juices

Ingredients for Energy and Stamina

Pre-workout juices are designed to provide a quick and efficient energy boost, helping to enhance stamina and endurance. These juices typically include ingredients rich in natural sugars, vitamins, and minerals that are easily absorbed by the body, offering immediate fuel for your workout. Beets, for example, are known to improve blood flow, while bananas provide a quick source of energy. Leafy greens like spinach and kale are packed with iron and vitamins, which help in sustaining energy levels and boosting overall performance.

Pre-Workout Juice Recipes

1. Beet Banana Boost

   - Ingredients:

     - 2 beetroots

     - 1 banana

     - 1 apple

- 1 handful of spinach

- 1 lemon (juiced)

- Instructions:

1. Wash all the ingredients thoroughly.

2. Peel the beetroots and banana.

3. Cut the beetroots, apple, and banana into pieces that will fit into your juicer.

4. Run the beetroots, banana, apple, and spinach through the juicer.

5. Stir in the lemon juice and serve immediately.

2. Green Power Juice

- Ingredients:

- 2 cups kale

- 1 cucumber

- 1 green apple

- 1-inch piece of ginger

- 1 lemon (juiced)

- Instructions:

1. Wash all the ingredients thoroughly.

2. Peel the cucumber and ginger.

3. Cut the cucumber and apple into chunks.

4. Run the kale, cucumber, apple, and ginger through the juicer.

5. Stir in the lemon juice and serve.

Post-Workout Recovery Juices

Ingredients for Recovery

Post-workout recovery juices focus on replenishing nutrients and aiding muscle repair. After an intense workout, your body needs specific nutrients to repair and build muscle tissue. These juices often contain ingredients rich in protein, antioxidants, and anti-inflammatory compounds to reduce muscle soreness and speed up recovery. Berries, for instance, are packed with antioxidants that help to combat oxidative stress, while bananas provide potassium, which is essential for muscle function. Leafy greens like spinach offer magnesium and vitamins that support muscle recovery.

Post-Workout Juice Recipes

1. Berry Banana Recovery

- Ingredients:

    - 1 cup mixed berries (strawberries, blueberries, raspberries)

    - 1 banana

    - 1 cup coconut water

    - 1 handful of spinach

- Instructions:

    1. Wash the berries and spinach thoroughly.

    2. Peel the banana.

    3. Combine the berries, banana, coconut water, and spinach in a blender.

    4. Blend until smooth.

    5. Serve immediately.

2. Pineapple Turmeric Refresher

    - Ingredients:

        - 1 cup pineapple chunks

        - 1 orange

        - 1-inch piece of turmeric root

        - 1 carrot

        - 1-inch piece of ginger

- Instructions:

    1. Wash all the ingredients thoroughly.

    2. Peel the orange, turmeric, and ginger.

    3. Cut the carrot into pieces.

    4. Run all ingredients through the juicer.

    5. Stir well and serve.

Hydration and Electrolyte Balance

Hydrating Ingredients

Staying hydrated is crucial, especially during and after physical activity. Hydrating juices often include ingredients high in water content and electrolytes, such as cucumber, watermelon, and coconut water. These ingredients help to replace lost fluids and maintain electrolyte balance, preventing dehydration and maintaining optimal body function. Cucumber and watermelon are particularly hydrating due to their high water content, while coconut water is rich in electrolytes like potassium, sodium, and magnesium, which are vital for maintaining fluid balance in the body.

Hydration Juice Recipes

1. Cucumber Watermelon Cooler

    - Ingredients:

- 1 cucumber

- 2 cups watermelon chunks

- 1 lemon (juiced)

- 1 handful of mint leaves

- Instructions:

1. Wash all the ingredients thoroughly.

2. Peel the cucumber if desired, and cut into chunks.

3. Combine the cucumber, watermelon, and mint leaves in a blender.

4. Blend until smooth.

5. Stir in the lemon juice and serve.

2. Coconut Citrus Hydrator

-Ingredients:

- 1 cup coconut water

- 1 orange

- 1 lime

- 1 lemon

- 1 tablespoon honey (optional)

- Instructions:

1. Peel the orange, lime, and lemon.

2. Combine the coconut water, orange, lime, and lemon in a blender.

3. Blend until smooth.

4. Add honey if desired for extra sweetness.

5. Serve chilled.

Chapter 5: Seasonal Juicing

Spring Juices

Seasonal Produce Guide

Spring is a season of renewal and growth, bringing an abundance of fresh and vibrant fruits and vegetables. During this time, you□llfind leafy greens like spinach, kale, and arugula, which are excellent for detoxifying the body. Herbs such as mint and parsley add a refreshing touch to juices. Spring also ushers in the sweetness of strawberries and the testiness of citrus fruits like lemons and oranges.

These ingredients help create refreshing and revitalizing juices, perfect for cleansing the body after the winter months and boosting overall vitality.

Spring Juice Recipes

1. Strawberry Mint Delight - Ingredients:

- 1 cup fresh strawberries

- 1 cucumber

- 1 handful of mint leaves

- 1 lemon (juiced)

- Instructions:

1. Wash all ingredients thoroughly.

2. Hull the strawberries and peel the cucumber if desired.

3. Blend the strawberries, cucumber, and mint leaves until smooth.

4. Stir in the lemon juice and serve immediately.

2. Green Spring Cleanse

- Ingredients:

- 2 cups spinach

- 1 green apple

- 1 cucumber

- 1 handful of parsley

- 1 lemon (juiced)

- Instructions:

1. Wash all ingredients thoroughly.

2. Core the apple and cut it into pieces.

3. Blend the spinach, apple, cucumber, and parsley until smooth.

4. Stir in the lemon juice and serve.

Summer Juices

Seasonal Produce Guide

Summer is the peak season for a wide variety of fruits and vegetables that are juicy, sweet, and hydrating. Produce like watermelon, cucumbers, berries, and tropical fruits such as mangoes and pineapples are at their best during this time. Additionally, summer herbs like basil and mint add a refreshing flavor to juices. These ingredients are perfect for creating cooling and hydrating juices that help to beat the heat and keep you refreshed.

Summer Juice Recipes

1. Watermelon Basil Cooler

  - Ingredients:

    - 2 cups watermelon chunks

    - 1 cucumber

    - 1 handful of basil leaves

    - 1 lime (juiced)

  - Instructions:

    1. Wash all ingredients thoroughly.

    2. Peel the cucumber if desired and cut into chunks.

    3. Blend the watermelon, cucumber, and basil leaves until smooth.

    4. Stir in the lime juice and serve chilled.

2. Tropical Berry Splash

  - Ingredients:

    - 1 cup mixed berries (strawberries, blueberries, raspberries)

    - 1 mango (peeled and pitted)

- 1 cup coconut water

- 1 handful of mint leaves

- Instructions:

1. Wash the berries and mint leaves thoroughly.

2. Blend the berries, mango, coconut water, and mint leaves until smooth.

3. Serve immediately for a refreshing summer treat.

THIS BLANK SPACE IS INTENTIONAL AND HAS BEEN DELIBERATELY INCLUDED TO ENHANCE THE READING EXPERIENCE. PLEASE CONTINUE WITH THE NEXT PAGE

Fall Juices

Seasonal Produce Guide

Fall brings a harvest of rich, hearty fruits and vegetables that are perfect for more grounding and warming juices. Apples, pears, carrots, and pumpkins are abundant in the fall, along with spices like ginger and cinnamon that add warmth. These ingredients are ideal for creating comforting and nourishing juices that help prepare the body for the colder months ahead.

Fall Juice Recipes

1. Apple Carrot Ginger Juice

   - Ingredients:

     - 2 apples

     - 3 carrots

     - 1-inch piece of ginger

     - 1 lemon (juiced)

   - Instructions:

     1. Wash all ingredients thoroughly.

     2. Core the apples and cut them into pieces.

3. Peel the carrots and ginger.

4. Blend the apples, carrots, and ginger until smooth.

5. Stir in the lemon juice and serve.

2. Pumpkin Spice Juice

   - Ingredients:

      - 1 cup pumpkin puree

      - 2 carrots

      - 1 orange (peeled)

      - 1/2 teaspoon cinnamon

      - 1/4 teaspoon nutmeg

   - Instructions:

      1. Wash the carrots thoroughly and peel them.

      2. Blend the pumpkin puree, carrots, and orange until smooth.

      3. Stir in the cinnamon and nutmeg.

      4. Serve chilled or slightly warmed.

Winter Juices

Seasonal Produce Guide

Winter is a time for robust and nutrient-dense produce that supports the immune system and provides warmth.

Citrus fruits like oranges, grapefruits, and lemons are in abundance, providing a rich source of vitamin C. Root vegetables like beets and carrots, along with greens like kale and spinach, are also in season, offering essential nutrients to keep you healthy during the colder months.

Winter Juice Recipes

1. Citrus Immunity Booster

   - Ingredients:

     - 2 oranges

     - 1 grapefruit

     - 1 lemon

     - 1-inch piece of ginger

   - Instructions:

     1. Peel the oranges, grapefruit, and lemon.

     2. Peel the ginger.

     3. Blend the citrus fruits and ginger until smooth.

     4. Serve immediately for a vitamin C boost.

2. Beet Carrot Kale Juice

   - Ingredients:

     - 2 beetroots

- 3 carrots

- 2 cups kale

- 1 apple

- 1 lemon (juiced)

- Instructions:

1. Wash all ingredients thoroughly.

2. Peel the beetroots and carrots.

3. Core the apple and cut it into pieces.

4. Blend the beetroots, carrots, kale, and apple until smooth.

5. Stir in the lemon juice and serve.

Chapter 6 : Advanced Juicing Techniques

Superfoods in Juices

Introduction to Superfoods

Superfoods are nutrient-rich ingredients that offer significant health benefits. Incorporating superfoods into your juices can amplify their nutritional value and provide an array of vitamins, minerals, antioxidants, and other beneficial compounds. Common superfoods include kale, spinach, berries, chia seeds, spirulina, and turmeric. These ingredients are known for their anti-inflammatory properties, high antioxidant content, and ability to boost immunity and overall health.

Superfood Juice Recipes

Kale Berry Blast

- Ingredients:

2 cups kale

1 cup mixed berries (blueberries, strawberries, raspberries)

1 banana

1 tablespoon chia seeds

1 cup coconut water

- Instructions:

1. Wash the kale and berries thoroughly.

2. Combine the kale, berries, banana, chia seeds, and coconut water in a blender.

3.Blend until smooth and serve immediately.

Spirulina Citrus Green Juice

- Ingredients:

2 cups spinach

1 green apple

1 orange (peeled)

1 teaspoon spirulina powder

1 lemon (juiced)

- Instructions:

1. Wash the spinach and apple thoroughly.

2. Core the apple and cut it into pieces.

3. Blend the spinach, apple, orange, and spirulina powder until smooth.

4. Stir in the lemon juice and serve.

Fermented Juices

Benefits of Fermentation

Fermentation is a process that uses natural bacteria to convert sugars into alcohol or acids, creating probiotic-rich beverages. Fermented juices, such as kombucha or kvass, are beneficial for gut health as they introduce healthy bacteria into the digestive system. These beverages can enhance digestion, boost the immune system, and improve overall health. The fermentation process also increases the bioavailability of nutrients, making it easier for the body to absorb vitamins and minerals.

Fermented Juice Recipes

Ginger Beet Kvass

- Ingredients:

2 large beets (peeled and chopped)

1-inch piece of ginger (sliced)

1 tablespoon sea salt

4 cups filtered water

- Instructions:

1. Place the beets and ginger in a large glass jar.

2. Dissolve the sea salt in filtered water and pour over the beets and ginger.

3. Cover the jar with a cloth and let it sit at room temperature for 3-5 days.

4. Strain and refrigerate before serving.

Citrus Kombucha

- Ingredients:

4 cups brewed black tea (cooled)

1/2 cup sugar

1 SCOBY (Symbiotic Culture of Bacteria and Yeast)

1 cup starter kombucha

1 orange (juiced)1 lemon (juiced)

- Instructions:

1. Brew the black tea and dissolve the sugar in it.

2. Let it cool to room temperature.

3. Pour the tea into a large glass jar and add the SCOBY and starter kombucha.

4. Cover the jar with a cloth and let it ferment at room temperature for 7-10 days.

After fermentation, remove the SCOBY and stir in the orange and lemon juice.

5. Refrigerate before serving.

Smoothies vs. Juices

Differences and Benefits

While both smoothies and juices are popular ways to consume fruits and vegetables, they have distinct differences. Juices are made by extracting the liquid from fruits and vegetables, leaving behind the fiber. This makes juices nutrient-dense and easy to digest, providing a quick energy boost and an immediate influx of vitamins and minerals. Smoothies, on the other hand, blend whole fruits and vegetables, including the fiber, which aids in digestion and keeps you fuller for longer. The choice between smoothies and juices depends on your nutritional needs and personal preferences.

When to Choose Each

Juices are ideal when you need a rapid infusion of nutrients, such as before or after workouts, or when you want to give your digestive system a break. They are also great for detoxifying the body. Smoothies are better suited for meal replacements or when you need sustained energy throughout the day. They are more filling and provide a balanced mix of macronutrients, including fiber, protein, and healthy fats.

Juicing and Fasting

Juicing can be a powerful tool when combined with fasting. Juice fasting involves consuming only fresh juices for a certain period, allowing the body to detoxify and reset. This practice can help with weight loss, improve digestion, and enhance mental clarity. However, it□s important to ensure that the juices consumed are nutrient-dense and balanced to provide the necessary vitamins and minerals during the fast.

Juicing and Clean Eating

Incorporating juicing into a clean eating regimen can significantly enhance your overall health. Clean eating focuses on consuming whole, unprocessed foods, and juicing provides an easy way to increase your intake of fruits and vegetables. Combining juicing with clean eating helps to flood your body with essential nutrients, improve digestion, boost energy levels, and support overall well-being. This holistic approach ensures that you are nourishing your body with high-quality, nutrient-dense foods.

Chapter 7: Juicing for Families

Juicing for Kids

Kid-Friendly Ingredients

When juicing for kids, it□simportant to choose ingredients that are not only nutritious but also appealing to young taste buds. Sweet fruits like apples, strawberries, and oranges are generally well-received by children. Adding vegetables such as carrots and cucumbers can increase the nutritional value without overpowering the sweetness. It□salso beneficial to involve kids in the juicing process, making is a fun and educational activity.

Fun and Nutritious Juice (popsicle) Recipes for Children

Sweet Carrot Apple Juice

- Ingredients:

2 apples

3 carrots

1 orange (peeled)

1 handful of spinach

- Instructions:

1. Wash all ingredients thoroughly.

2.Core the apples and peel the carrots and orange.

3. Blend the apples, carrots, orange, and spinach until smooth.

4. Serve immediately for a sweet and nutritious treat.

Berry Banana Smoothie

- Ingredients:

1 cup mixed berries (strawberries, blueberries, raspberries)

1 banana

1 cup yogurt

1/2 cup orange juice

- Instructions:

1. Wash the berries thoroughly.

2. Combine the berries, banana, yogurt, and orange juice in a blender.

3. Blend until smooth and serve.

Juicing for Seniors

Nutrients for Aging

As we age, our nutritional needs change, and it becomes increasingly important to consume foods that support overall health and vitality. Juices can be an excellent way for seniors to obtain essential nutrients, especially if they have difficulty chewing or digesting solid foods. Ingredients rich in antioxidants, vitamins, and minerals such as berries, leafy greens, and citrus fruits are particularly beneficial. Adding anti-inflammatory ingredients like turmeric and ginger can also help manage age-related conditions.

Senior-Friendly Juice Recipes

Anti-Inflammatory Green Juice

- Ingredients:

2 cups kale

1 cucumber

1 green apple

1-inch piece of turmeric

1 lemon (juiced)

- Instructions:

1. Wash all ingredients thoroughly.

2. Peel the cucumber and turmeric.

3. Core the apple and cut it into pieces.

4. Blend the kale, cucumber, apple, and turmeric until smooth.

5. Stir in the lemon juice and serve.

Citrus Berry Boost

- Ingredients:

1 cup mixed berries (strawberries, blueberries, raspberries)

1 orange (peeled)

1/2 cup pomegranate juice

1 tablespoon flaxseeds

Instructions:

1. Wash the berries thoroughly.

2. Combine the berries, orange, pomegranate juice, and flaxseeds in a blender.

3. Blend until smooth and serve.

Chapter 8: Troubleshooting and FAQs

Common Juicing Problems

Bitter or Unpleasant Tastes

Bitterness in juice can often be attributed to certain ingredients like citrus peels or dark leafy greens such as kale or collard greens. To mitigate bitterness, try adding sweeter fruits like apples, oranges, or berries to balance the flavor. Additionally, incorporating herbs like mint or basil can add freshness and reduce bitterness. Adjusting the ratio of bitter to sweet ingredients and experimenting with different combinations can help create a more palatable juice.

Separation and Settling

Juice separation occurs naturally due to the varying densities of ingredients. Ingredients like citrus juices and watermelon tend to separate quickly. To minimize separation, stir the juice thoroughly before serving or storing. Adding a small amount of citrus juice or using a high-powered blender can also help emulsify the juice and reduce settling over time. Remember that some settling is normal, and shaking or stirring before consumption can remix the flavors.

Frequently Asked Questions

How Much Juice Should I Drink?

The amount of juice you should drink depends on your individual needs and goals. As a general guideline, consuming one to two cups of fresh juice per day can provide essential nutrients without overwhelming your system. It□simportant to balance juice consumption with a variety of other nutritious foods to maintain a well-rounded diet.

Can I Store Juice Overnight?

Ideally, it's best to consume juice immediately after preparation to retain maximum freshness and nutritional value. However, if you need to store juice, place it in an airtight container in the refrigerator immediately after juicing. Juice can typically be stored for up to 24-48 hours, although it may begin to lose some nutrients and freshness over time. Shake or stir the juice well before drinking if it separates.

What About Pulp?

Pulp contains dietary fiber and other beneficial nutrients that may be lost during juicing. Some people choose to incorporate pulp back into their diet by adding it to smoothies, soups, or baked goods. Alternatively, you can use a juicer with a pulp extractor to retain more fiber in your juice. Experiment with different uses for pulp to find what works best for your preferences and nutritional needs.

Common Juicing beginners ask

1. How can I reduce foaming in my juices?

 Ans: Foaming can occur due to certain ingredients or the juicing process itself. To minimize foaming, try adding ingredients slowly and avoid overfilling the juicer chute. Skimming off foam with a spoon or letting the juice settle before pouring can also help.

2. Can I juice citrus fruits with their peel?

  Ans: Yes, citrus peels contain valuable nutrients, but they can impart a bitter flavor to the juice. If juicing citrus with peel, ensure the fruit is thoroughly washed to remove any residues or pesticides.

3. What are some tips for juicing on a budget?

Ans: To juice economically, focus on seasonal produce and buy in bulk when possible. Use cheaper base ingredients like carrots or apples and supplement with smaller amounts of more expensive items like leafy greens or berries.

4. Is it necessary to buy an expensive juicer?

 Ans: The price of juicers can vary widely, but a quality juicer doesn't always have to be expensive. Consider your juicing habits and preferences (such as ease of cleaning, juicing efficiency) when choosing a juicer that fits your budget and needs.

5. How can I make my juices more filling?

Ans: Adding ingredients high in fiber and protein, such as chia seeds, flaxseeds, or Greek yogurt, can increase the satiety of your juices. Alternatively, consider incorporating juiced vegetables that are naturally more filling, like celery or cucumber.

Chapter 9: Juicing Recipes Collection

Fruit Juices

Explore a variety of pure fruit juice recipes that highlight the natural sweetness and flavors of fruits.

Recipes

1. Classic Citrus Blast

Ingredients

- 2 oranges, peeled

- 1 grapefruit, peeled

- 1 lemon, peeled

Instructions

- Wash all fruits thoroughly.

- Peel the oranges, grapefruit, and lemon.

- Juice all ingredients together.

- Stir well and serve over ice for a refreshing citrus burst.

2. Tropical Paradise

Ingredients:

  - 1 cup pineapple chunks

  - 1 banana

  - 1/2 cup mango chunks

  - 1/2 cup coconut water

Instructions:

  - Prepare all fruits by washing and cutting into chunks.

  - Blend pineapple, banana, mango, and coconut water until smooth.

  - Pour into a glass and enjoy the tropical flavors.

3. Berry Berry Blast

Ingredients:

  - 1 cup strawberries

  - 1 cup blueberries

  - 1 cup raspberries

  - 1 tablespoon honey (optional for added sweetness)

Instructions:

- Wash berries thoroughly.

- Blend all berries together until smooth.

- Taste and add honey if desired.

- Serve chilled for a delightful berry treat.

Vegetable Juices

Discover vegetable juice recipes that are packed with essential vitamins, minerals, and antioxidants.

Recipes:

1. Garden Greens Delight

Ingredients:

  - 2 cups spinach

  - 1 cucumber

  - 2 celery stalks

  - 1 green apple

  - 1 lemon, peeled

Instructions:

  - Wash all vegetables and fruit.

  - Cut cucumber and celery into smaller pieces.

  - Juice spinach, cucumber, celery, apple, and lemon.

  - Stir well and serve immediately for a nutrient-packed green juice.

2. Carrot Ginger Energizer

Ingredients:

  - 4 carrots

  - 1-inch piece of ginger

  - 1 orange, peeled

Instructions:

  - Wash and peel carrots and ginger.

  - Peel orange.

  - Juice carrots, ginger, and orange together.

  - Stir and enjoy the zesty carrot ginger juice.

3. Beetroot Power Punch

Ingredients:

  - 2 beetroots, peeled and chopped

  - 1 cucumber

  - 2 stalks of kale

  - 1 apple

Instructions:

- Wash all vegetables and fruit thoroughly.

- Cut cucumber and apple into smaller pieces.

- Juice beetroots, cucumber, kale, and apple together.

- Mix well and serve over ice for a vibrant beetroot juice.

Mixed Juices

Enjoy creative combinations of fruits and vegetables in these mixed juice recipes that offer a balance of flavors and nutrients.

Recipes:

1. Pineapple Cucumber Cooler

Ingredients:

- 1 cup pineapple chunks

- 1 cucumber

- 1 lime, peeled

Instructions:

- Wash and prepare all ingredients.

- Peel cucumber and lime.

- Juice pineapple, cucumber, and lime together.

- Stir and serve chilled for a refreshing tropical mix.

2. Apple Berry Bliss

Ingredients:

  - 1 apple

  - 1 cup mixed berries (strawberries, blueberries, raspberries)

  - 1/2 cup water

Instructions:

- Wash all fruits thoroughly.

- Core the apple and cut into chunks.

- Blend apple, mixed berries, and water until smooth.

- Pour into a glass and enjoy the fruity goodness.

Herbal and Spiced Juices

 Experience the added benefits of herbs and spices in these flavorful juice recipes that support various health goals.

Recipes:

1. Minty Watermelon Refresher

Ingredients:

  - 2 cups watermelon, cubed

  - 1 cucumber

  - 1 handful of fresh mint leaves

Instructions:

  - Wash all ingredients.

  - Cut watermelon and cucumber into chunks.

  - Juice watermelon, cucumber, and mint together.

  - Stir and serve over ice for a cooling summer drink.

2. Spicy Turmeric Carrot Juice

Ingredients:

- 4 carrots

- 1-inch piece of fresh turmeric root

- 1 orange, peeled

Instructions:

- Wash and peel carrots and turmeric root.

- Peel orange.

- Juice carrots, turmeric root, and orange together.

- Mix well and enjoy the warming flavors of turmeric and carrot.

These recipes provide a variety of options for different tastes and health goals, showcasing the versatility and deliciousness of juicing with fruits, vegetables, herbs, and spices.

Chapter 10: Juicing as a Lifestyle

Integrating Juicing into Daily Life

Routine and Habit Building:

Integrating juicing into your daily life begins with establishing a routine and building healthy habits. Choose a consistent time each day that works best for you—whether it's in the morning to kickstart your day or in the evening as a relaxing wind-down ritual. By making juicing a regular part of your schedule, you'll create a habit that enhances your overall well-being. Set up your juicing station for convenience, keep your favorite ingredients stocked, and enjoy the process of preparing fresh juices that nourish both body and mind.

Meal Planning with Juices:

Meal planning with juices is a practical way to ensure you get a variety of nutrients throughout the day. Incorporate juices as part of your balanced diet by planning recipes that complement your meals. Consider juices that align with your nutritional needs and tastes, whether it's a green detox blend to start your day or a hydrating fruit juice as an afternoon pick-me-up. By including juices in your meal planning, you'll optimize your nutrient intake and maintain a healthy lifestyle effortlessly.

Juicing on the Go: Travel Tips

Portable Juicing Solutions:

Maintaining your juicing routine while traveling is made easier with portable solutions. Invest in a compact, travel-friendly juicer or blender that fits into your suitcase or carry-on. Prepare single-serving juice packs in advance by pre-cutting fruits and vegetables that travel well. Look for local markets or grocery stores at your destination to replenish fresh produce. Whether you're on a business trip or vacation, portable juicing solutions ensure you can continue to enjoy fresh, nutrient-rich juices wherever your travels take you.

Community and Sharing

Joining Juicing Communities:

Connecting with juicing communities provides support, inspiration, and valuable insights into juicing practices. Engage with like-minded individuals through online forums, social media groups, or local meet-ups to share recipes, tips, and experiences. Joining juicing communities not only expands your knowledge but also motivates you to explore new ingredients and techniques, enhancing your juicing journey.

Hosting Juicing Parties:

Hosting juicing parties is a fun way to introduce friends and family to the benefits of juicing. Plan themed gatherings where everyone can participate in juicing together and experiment with different recipes. Whether it's a citrus-themed brunch or a green juice tasting, hosting juicing parties fosters a sense of community and encourages healthy habits among your social circle. Share your passion for juicing, exchange creative ideas, and enjoy the delicious and nutritious juices you create together.

Embracing juicing as a lifestyle involves integrating it into your daily routines, adapting it to your travel adventures, and connecting with others who share your passion. By making juicing a regular part of your life and engaging with a supportive community, you'll enhance your well-being and enjoy the journey towards a healthier lifestyle.

Chapter 11: Juicing for Mental Clarity and Mood

Mental clarity and mood balance are essential components of overall well-being. With the right combination of nutrients, juices can significantly impact brain health, cognitive function, and emotional balance. This chapter delves into the benefits of specific ingredients and provides recipes to enhance brain health and improve mood.

Juices for Brain Health

Ingredients for Cognitive Function

Certain fruits, vegetables, and herbs are known for their cognitive-enhancing properties. These ingredients provide essential vitamins, minerals, antioxidants, and other compounds that support brain health and cognitive function:

- Blueberries: Rich in antioxidants, particularly flavonoids, which have been shown to improve memory and cognitive function.

- Spinach: High in lutein, folate, beta carotene, and other antioxidants that support brain health.

- Avocado: Contains healthy fats that promote blood flow to the brain.

- Beets: High in nitrates, which improve blood flow to the brain, enhancing cognitive function.

- Turmeric: Contains curcumin, known for its anti-inflammatory and antioxidant properties, which support brain health.

- Walnuts: Rich in omega-3 fatty acids, which are essential for brain function.

~ Brain-Boosting Juice Recipes

1. Blueberry Brain Booster

  - 1 cup blueberries

  - 1 cup spinach

  - 1/2 avocado

  - 1/2 cucumber

  - 1/2 lemon (peeled)

  - 1-inch piece of ginger

  - Water or coconut water as needed

Blend all ingredients until smooth. Enjoy this refreshing juice to give your brain a boost.

2. Beet and Berry Cognitive Enhancer

  - 1 medium beet (peeled and chopped)

  - 1 cup mixed berries (blueberries, strawberries, raspberries)

  - 1 apple (cored and chopped)

  - 1/2 lemon (peeled)

  - 1-inch piece of turmeric

Instruction:

  1. Juice all ingredients together and stir well.

 This vibrant juice supports blood flow to the brain, enhancing cognitive function.

~ Mood-Enhancing Juices

Ingredients for Emotional Balance

To improve mood and emotional balance, look for ingredients rich in vitamins, minerals, and compounds that support neurotransmitter function and reduce inflammation:

- Bananas: High in vitamin B6, which helps produce serotonin, the "feel-good" hormone.

- Oranges: Rich in vitamin C, which can reduce stress and improve mood.

- Kale: Contains magnesium, which plays a role in brain health and mood regulation.

- Carrots: High in beta carotene, which supports overall brain function.

- Ginger: Has anti-inflammatory properties that can help reduce symptoms of anxiety and depression.

- Chamomile: Known for its calming effects, chamomile can help reduce anxiety and improve sleep quality.

Mood-Enhancing Juice Recipes

1. Banana Citrus Uplift

   - 1 banana

   - 2 oranges (peeled)

   - 1 carrot (peeled and chopped)

   - 1 handful of kale

   - 1-inch piece of ginger

Instruction:

S 1. Blend all ingredients until smooth.

This juice is perfect for boosting your mood and keeping stress at bay.

2. Calm and Happy Chamomile Blend

   - 1 apple (cored and chopped)

   - 1 pear (cored and chopped)

   - 1/2 cucumber

   - 1 handful of spinach

   - 1 chamomile tea bag (brewed and cooled)

   - 1 teaspoon honey (optional)

Instructions:

   1. Juice the apple, pear, cucumber, and spinach together.

2. Mix in the cooled chamomile tea and honey.

This soothing juice helps promote relaxation and a positive mood. Incorporating juices into your daily routine can have profound effects on your mental clarity and mood. By selecting ingredients that support cognitive function and emotional balance, you can create delicious and nutritious juices that contribute to overall mental well-being. Try these recipes and experiment with your own combinations to find the perfect blends for your brain and mood health.

THIS BLANK SPACE IS INTENTIONAL AND HAS BEEN DELIBERATELY INCLUDED TO ENHANCE THE READING EXPERIENCE. PLEASE CONTINUE WITH THE NEXT PAGE.

Chapter 12: Juicing for Specific Diets

Juicing can be adapted to fit various dietary lifestyles and needs, offering a versatile way to ensure you receive essential nutrients while adhering to specific dietary guidelines. This chapter explores juicing options for vegans, vegetarians, those following Paleo and Keto diets, and individuals requiring gluten-free options.

Juicing for Vegans and Vegetarians

Plant-Based Juice Recipes

Vegans and vegetarians often focus on maximizing nutrient intake from plant sources. Juicing is an excellent way to concentrate these nutrients and enjoy a variety of fruits and vegetables in a convenient form.

1. Green Power Juice

   - 1 cup kale

   - 1 cup spinach

   - 1 cucumber

   - 2 green apples (cored)

- 1 lemon (peeled)

- 1-inch piece of ginger

Juice all ingredients together for a refreshing, nutrient-dense drink packed with vitamins A, C, K, and iron.

2. Tropical Carrot Delight

- 4 carrots

- 1 mango (peeled and pitted)

- 1 orange (peeled)

- 1/2 inch piece of turmeric

This juice is rich in beta-carotene, vitamin C, and antioxidants, perfect for boosting immune health.

Paleo and Keto Juices

Low-Carb Juice Recipes

The Paleo and Keto diets emphasize low-carb, high-fat, and moderate-protein intake. Juicing for these diets requires careful selection of low-sugar fruits and vegetables.

1. Avocado Green Juice

  - 1/2 avocado

  - 1 cup spinach

  - 1 cucumber

  - 1 celery stalk

  - 1/2 lemon (peeled)

  - Water as needed

Blend the avocado separately and combine with the juice of other ingredients. This low-carb, high-fat juice is rich in healthy fats and electrolytes.

2. Cucumber and Mint Refresher

  - 2 cucumbers

  - 1 handful of fresh mint leaves

  - 1 lime (peeled)

This hydrating juice is low in carbs and helps with hydration and electrolyte balance, perfect for Paleo and Keto followers.

Gluten-Free Juices

Safe Ingredients for Celiacs

For individuals with celiac disease or gluten sensitivity, it's crucial to ensure that all ingredients are free from gluten contamination. Fresh fruits, vegetables, and herbs are naturally gluten-free, but always verify the sources if you are purchasing pre-cut or packaged produce.

Gluten-Free Juice Recipes

1. Berry Citrus Blast

   - 1 cup strawberries

   - 1 cup blueberries

   - 1 orange (peeled)

   - 1/2 lemon (peeled)

   - 1 cup coconut water

This vibrant juice is packed with antioxidants, vitamin C, and hydration, all from naturally gluten-free ingredients.

2. Pineapple Ginger Cleanse

- 1/2 pineapple (peeled and cored)

- 1 cucumber

- 1-inch piece of ginger

- 1 handful of parsley

Combining anti-inflammatory ginger and detoxifying parsley, this juice is excellent for digestion and overall wellness.

Juicing offers a flexible way to accommodate various dietary preferences and requirements. Whether you're vegan, vegetarian, following a Paleo or Keto diet, or need to avoid gluten, there are plenty of delicious and nutritious juice options available. By selecting the right ingredients, you can enjoy the benefits of juicing while staying true to your dietary goals. Experiment with these recipes and create your own to fit your specific diet and taste preferences.

Chapter 13: Juicing for Beauty and Anti-Aging

Juicing can be an effective way to nourish your skin, hair, and nails from the inside out. By incorporating specific ingredients known for their anti-aging properties, you can help maintain a youthful appearance and support overall beauty.

Anti-Aging Ingredients

Nutrients for Youthful Skin

Collagen-Boosting Foods: Ingredients like citrus fruits (rich in vitamin C) help boost collagen production, essential for skin elasticity.

Antioxidant-Rich Foods: Berries, pomegranates, and spinach contain antioxidants that protect against free radicals and skin aging.

Hydrating Ingredients: Cucumbers and aloe vera keep the skin hydrated and plump.Omega-3 Fatty Acids: Flaxseeds and walnuts provide essential fatty acids that maintain skin barrier function and reduce inflammation.

Anti-Aging Juice Recipes

Radiant Skin Elixir

-1 cucumber

-1 cup spinach

-1 apple

-1/2 lemon (peeled)

- 1-inch piece of aloe vera gel

Juice all ingredients together. This hydrating and collagen-boosting juice is perfect for maintaining a youthful glow.

Berry Antioxidant Blast

-1 cup mixed berries (blueberries, strawberries, raspberries)1 pomegranate (seeds only)1 orange (peeled)

-1 teaspoon flaxseed oil

This juice is packed with antioxidants and omega-3s, crucial for combating skin aging and promoting healthy skin.

Hair and Nail Health

Ingredients for Strength and Shine

Biotin-Rich Foods: Ingredients like sweet potatoes and spinach are rich in biotin, which supports hair and nail growth.

Silica-Rich Foods: Cucumbers and bell peppers contain silica, which strengthens hair and nails.

Protein Sources: Nuts and seeds provide the necessary protein for strong hair and nails.

Beauty-Enhancing Juice Recipes

Shiny Hair Juice

-1 sweet potato (peeled)

-1 bell pepper

-1 handful of spinach

-1/2 apple

Juice all ingredients for a biotin and silica-rich drink that promotes strong, shiny hair.

Nail Strengthener

-1 cucumber

-1 cup kale1 carrot

-1 handful of almonds (blended separately and added)

This juice provides essential nutrients to support nail health and strength.

Chapter 14: Juicing for Stress Relief and Relaxation

Juicing can also play a role in stress management and relaxation. By selecting ingredients known for their calming properties, you can create juices that help reduce anxiety and promote a sense of calm. Ingredients for Relaxation.

Calming Herbs and Fruits

Chamomile: Known for its calming effects, chamomile can help reduce anxiety. Lavender: Has soothing properties that can help alleviate stress.

Lemon Balm: A calming herb that can reduce anxiety and promote relaxation. Fruits: Bananas, which contain tryptophan, a precursor to serotonin, can improve mood. Stress-Relief Juice Recipes

Calming Chamomile Citrus

-1 chamomile tea bag (brewed and cooled)

-2 oranges (peeled)

-1 banana

-1/2 lemon (peeled)

Blend the banana and combine with the juice of the other ingredients and chamomile tea. This soothing juice helps calm the nerves.

Lavender Lemonade

,-1 teaspoon dried lavender (steeped in hot water and cooled)

-1 lemon (peeled)

-1 apple

-1/2 cucumber

Juice the lemon, apple, and cucumber, then mix with the cooled lavender tea. This refreshing juice has a calming effect on the mind.

Bedtime Juices

Sleep-Promoting Ingredients

Tart Cherry Juice: Contains melatonin, which can help regulate sleep. Kiwi: Rich in serotonin, which helps with sleep.

Almonds: Contain magnesium, which promotes sleep.

Relaxing Juice Recipes for Better Sleep

Cherry Sleep Aid

-1 cup tart cherries

-1 kiwi (peeled)

-1/2 banana

Blend all ingredients for a melatonin-rich drink that promotes a good night's sleep.

Almond Kiwi Nightcap

-1 handful of almonds (blended separately and added)

-2 kiwis (peeled)

-1 apple

Juice the kiwis and apple, then mix with the blended almonds.

This juice is rich in magnesium and serotonin to help you relax and sleep well.

Chapter 15: Economic and Sustainable Juicing

Juicing can be made economical and sustainable by choosing affordable ingredients and adopting practices that reduce waste.

Budget-Friendly Juicing

Affordable Ingredients

Carrots: Inexpensive and rich in beta-carotene.

Apples: Affordable and versatile.

Cucumbers: Hydrating and budget-friendly.

Spinach: Inexpensive and nutrient-dense.

Cost-Effective Juice Recipes

Simple Carrot Delight

-4 carrots

-1 apple

-1/2 lemon (peeled)

This juice is affordable and packed with vitamins and antioxidants.

Cucumber Spinach Refresh

-1 cucumber

-1 handful of spinach

-1 apple

A hydrating and nutrient-rich juice that won't break the bank.

Sustainable Juicing Practices

Reducing Waste

Use the Pulp: Incorporate leftover pulp into recipes like muffins, soups, or compost it.

Buy Local and Seasonal: Local produce is fresher, often cheaper, and has a lower environmental impact.

Reusable Bags and Containers: Reduce plastic use by opting for reusable options. Eco-Friendly Juicing Tips Compost Scraps: Composting fruit and vegetable scraps reduces waste and enriches the soil.

Grow Your Own: Growing your own herbs and some vegetables can be economical and sustainable.

s

Chapter 16: Juicing for Athletes and High-Performance Individuals

Juicing can provide essential nutrients for athletes and those seeking to enhance their physical performance.

High-Performance Ingredients

Ingredients for Peak Performance

Beets: Improve blood flow and endurance.

Spinach: High in iron, supporting oxygen transport in the blood. Bananas: Provide quick energy from natural sugars and potassium to prevent capsica Seeds: Rich in omega-3s and protein.

Athlete-Focused Juice Recipes

Beet Performance Boost

-2 beets

-1 apple

-1 carrot

This juice enhances endurance and improves blood flow, perfect for athletes.

Banana Spinach Power

-1 banana

-1 cup spinach

-1 apple

- 1 tablespoon chia seeds (blended separately and added)

This juice provides energy and essential nutrients for peak performance. Recovery and Muscle Repair

Post-Exercise Ingredients

Pineapple: Contains bromelain, which reduces inflammation. Ginger: Anti-inflammatory properties aid in recovery.

Coconut Water: Hydrates and replenishes electrolytes. Berries: Antioxidants aid in muscle repair.

Recovery Juice Recipes

Hydration Power Juice

This juice is perfect for replenishing lost fluids and electrolytes after a workout.

Ingredients:

1 cucumber

2 celery stalks

1/2 cup coconut water

1/2 lemon (peeled)

1 apple (optional for sweetness)

A pinch of sea salt (optional for extra electrolytes)

Instructions:

Wash all the ingredients.

Peel the lemon.

Cut the cucumber, apple, and celery into pieces that fit your juicer.

Juice all the ingredients together.

Stir in coconut water and sea salt, then drink immediately.

 Anti-Inflammatory Recovery Juice

Packed with anti-inflammatory ingredients, this juice helps reduce muscle soreness and speed up recovery.

Ingredients:

1 pineapple (peeled and chopped)

2 carrots

1 orange (peeled)

1/2 inch piece of ginger

1/2 inch piece of turmeric root (or 1/2 teaspoon turmeric powder)

1/2 lemon (peeled)

Instructions:

Wash all the ingredients.

Peel the orange, lemon, ginger, and turmeric root.

Cut the pineapple, carrots, and ginger into pieces that fit your juicer.

Juice all the ingredients together.

Stir and drink fresh to benefit from the anti-inflammatory properties.

Muscle Recovery Juice

This juice supports muscle repair with a good balance of vitamins and minerals, helping you recover faster.

Ingredients:

1 beetroot (peeled)

2 carrots

1 apple

1/2 cucumber

1/2 inch piece of ginger

1/2 lemon (peeled)

Instructions:

Wash all the ingredients.

Peel the beetroot, lemon, and ginger.

Cut the beetroot, carrots, apple, and cucumber into pieces that fit your juicer.

Juice everything together.

Stir and drink immediately after your workout.

Energy Boost Juice

This juice is ideal for replenishing glycogen stores and giving you a quick energy boost after a workout.

Ingredients:

1 banana (blended, not juiced)

1/2 cup pineapple chunks

1 orange (peeled)

1/2 cup almond milk or coconut water

1 tablespoon chia seeds (for added protein and fiber)

Instructions:

Peel and chop the banana and orange.

Juice the pineapple and orange.

Blend the juice with the banana, almond milk, and chia seeds until smooth.

Drink immediately for a refreshing energy boost.

Replenishing Green Juice

This juice is loaded with greens to restore vitamins and minerals depleted during your workout.

Ingredients:

1 handful of spinach

1 handful of kale

1 green apple

1/2 cucumber

1/2 lemon (peeled)

1/2 inch piece of ginger

Instructions:

Wash all the ingredients.

Peel the lemon and ginger.

Cut the cucumber and apple into pieces that fit your juicer.

Juice the greens first, followed by the apple, cucumber, lemon, and ginger.

Stir and drink immediately to replenish your body.

Protein-Packed Recovery Juice

Ideal for muscle recovery, this juice combines protein and carbs for a balanced post-workout drink.

Ingredients:

1 banana (blended, not juiced)

1/2 cup Greek yogurt or a plant-based protein powder

1/2 cup almond milk or coconut water

1/2 cup blueberries

1 handful of spinach

Instructions:

Blend the banana, Greek yogurt or protein powder, almond milk, blueberries, and spinach together.

Blend until smooth and drink immediately after your workout to help with muscle recovery.

THIS BLANK SPACE IS INTENTIONAL AND HAS BEEN DELIBERATELY INCLUDED TO ENHANCE THE READING EXPERIENCE. PLEASE CONTINUE WITH THE NEXT PAGE.

Chapter 17: Cultural and Global Juicing Traditions

Juices From Around The World

Juicing is a global practice with unique traditions and recipes from different cultures. Exploring these can offer new flavors and nutritional benefits. Juices from Around the World Cultural Ingredients and Recipes

Aloe Vera Juice (Middle East): Known for its hydrating and digestive properties. Agua Fresca (Mexico): A refreshing juice made with various fruits. Lassi (India): A yogurt-based drink, often with added fruits and spices.

Global Juicing Traditions

Middle Eastern Aloe Vera Juice

-1 cup aloe vera gel

-1 cucumber

-1 lemon (peeled)

-1 tablespoon honey (optional)

This juice is hydrating and soothing for the digestive system.

Mexican Agua Fresca

-1 cup watermelon (cubed)

- 1 lime (peeled)

-1 cup water

-1 teaspoon sugar (optional)

Blend all ingredients and strain. This refreshing juice is perfect for hot days. Fusion Juicing

Combining Global Flavors

Thai-Inspired Coconut Lemongrass Juice: Combining tropical flavors with a touch of spice.

Mediterranean Citrus Herb Juice: Using herbs like mint and basil with citrus fruits.

Coconut Lemongrass Delight

1 cup coconut water

1 stalk lemongrass (chopped)

1 lime (peeled)

1/2 pineapple (peeled and cored)

1 teaspoon honey (optional)

Blend all ingredients until smooth and strain if desired. This juice combines tropical sweetness with a refreshing hint of lemongrass.

Mediterranean Citrus Herb Juice

1 orange (peeled)

1 lemon (peeled)1 handful of fresh mint leaves1 handful of fresh basil leaves1 cucumber Juice the citrus fruits and cucumber together, then blend with mint and basil for a fragrant and invigorating drink.

Sure! Here are the recipes separated for easy copying and pasting:

Agua de Jamaica (Mexico)

Ingredients:

- 1 cup dried hibiscus flowers

- 4 cups water

- 1/2 cup sugar (or to taste)

- Ice cubes

Instructions:

1. Bring 4 cups of water to a boil.

2. Add the dried hibiscus flowers and reduce the heat.

3. Let it simmer for about 10 minutes.

4. Remove from heat and strain the flowers.

5. Add sugar and stir until dissolved.

6. Let it cool, then serve over ice.

Mango Lassi (India)

Ingredients:

- 1 ripe mango, peeled and chopped

- 1 cup plain yogurt

- 1/2 cup milk

- 1-2 tablespoons sugar (optional)

- A pinch of cardamom powder (optional)

- Ice cubes

Instructions:

1. Combine mango, yogurt, milk, and sugar in a blender.

2. Blend until smooth and creamy.

3. Add cardamom powder if desired.

4. Serve chilled with ice cubes.

Bissap (West Africa)

Ingredients:

- 1 cup dried hibiscus flowers

- 4 cups water

- 1/2 cup sugar (or to taste)

- 1 tablespoon grated ginger (optional)

- Mint leaves (optional)

- Ice cubes

Instructions:

1. Boil 4 cups of water and add hibiscus flowers.

2. Let it simmer for 10 minutes.

3. Add grated ginger if desired.

4. Strain the liquid into a jug.

5. Add sugar and stir until dissolved.

6. Let it cool, then serve with ice and mint leaves.

Chicha Morada (Peru)

Ingredients:

- 1 cup purple corn kernels

- 4 cups water

- 1 cinnamon stick

- 4 cloves

- 1/2 pineapple, peeled and chopped

- 1/4 cup sugar (or to taste)

- Juice of 1 lime

- Ice cubes

Instructions:

1. In a pot, combine purple corn, water, cinnamon, cloves, and pineapple.

2. Bring to a boil and then simmer for 45 minutes.

3. Strain the liquid into a jug.

4. Add sugar and lime juice, stirring until sugar dissolves.

5. Let it cool, then serve over ice.

Ayran (Turkey)

Ingredients:

- 1 cup plain yogurt

- 1/2 cup cold water

- A pinch of salt

- Ice cubes

Instructions:

1. Whisk yogurt, water, and salt together until smooth.

2. Adjust salt to taste.

3. Serve chilled with ice cubes.

Tejuino (Mexico)

Ingredients:

- 1 cup corn masa dough

- 4 cups water

- 1/2 cup piloncillo (or brown sugar)

- Juice of 2 limes

- Salt to taste

- Ice cubes

Instructions:

1. Dissolve the masa in water and bring to a boil.

2. Reduce the heat and let it simmer until it thickens.

3. Add piloncillo and stir until dissolved.

4. Let it cool, then add lime juice and salt.

5. Serve over ice with a pinch of salt.

Ribena (United Kingdom)

Ingredients:

- 2 cups blackcurrants

- 4 cups water

- 1/2 cup sugar (or to taste)

Instructions:

1. Boil blackcurrants in water for about 10 minutes.

2. Strain the mixture to remove the pulp.

3. Return the liquid to the pot and add sugar.

4. Simmer until the sugar is dissolved.

5. Let it cool, then serve chilled.

Es Teler (Indonesia)

Ingredients:

- 1 ripe avocado, diced

- 1 cup young coconut meat, sliced

- 1 cup jackfruit, sliced

- 1/2 cup sweetened condensed milk

- 1/2 cup coconut milk

- Ice cubes

Instructions:

1. In a large bowl, combine avocado, coconut meat, and jackfruit.

2. Mix in sweetened condensed milk and coconut milk.

3. Serve in a glass over ice.

Qamar al-Din (Middle East)

Ingredients:

- 200g dried apricot paste

- 4 cups water

- 1/4 cup sugar (or to taste)

- Ice cubes

Instructions:

1. Cut the apricot paste into small pieces.

2. Soak the pieces in water overnight or for at least 4 hours.

3. Blend the mixture until smooth.

4. Add sugar and stir until dissolved.

5. Serve chilled with ice.

Suco de Caju (Brazil)

Ingredients:

- 1 cashew fruit (caju), chopped

- 1/2 cup water

- 1-2 tablespoons sugar (optional)

- Ice cubes

Instructions:

1. Blend the cashew fruit with water until smooth.

2. Strain the juice to remove any pulp.

3. Add sugar if desired.

4. Serve chilled over ice.

Sujeonggwa (Korea)

Ingredients:

- 4 cups water

- 2 cinnamon sticks

- 1/4 cup sliced ginger

- 1/2 cup dried persimmons

- 1/4 cup sugar (or to taste)

- Pine nuts for garnish

Instructions:

1. Boil water with cinnamon sticks and ginger for 20 minutes.

2. Remove from heat and add dried persimmons and sugar.

3. Let it cool, then chill in the refrigerator.

4. Serve cold with pine nuts on top.

Ampalaya Juice (Philippines)

Ingredients:

- 1 bitter melon (ampalaya), seeds removed and chopped

- 1 cup water

- 1-2 tablespoons honey or sugar

Instructions:

1. Blend the bitter melon with water until smooth.

2. Strain the juice to remove the pulp.

3. Add honey or sugar to taste.

4. Serve chilled.

Aloe Vera Juice (Global)

Ingredients:

- 1 aloe vera leaf

- 1 cup water

- 1 tablespoon lemon juice

- 1-2 tablespoons honey

Instructions:

1. Cut the aloe vera leaf and scoop out the gel.

2. Blend the gel with water, lemon juice, and honey.

3. Strain the mixture if desired.

4. Serve chilled.

Seco (Ecuador)

Ingredients:

- 2 naranjillas (lulo), peeled and chopped

- 1/2 cup water

- 1-2 tablespoons sugar

- A pinch of cinnamon (optional)

- Ice cubes

Instructions:

1. Blend the naranjillas with water until smooth.

2. Strain the juice to remove the pulp.

3. Add sugar and cinnamon if desired.

4. Serve chilled over ice.

Moro Blood Orange Juice (Italy)

Ingredients:

- 4-6 Moro blood oranges

Instructions:

1. Peel the blood oranges.

2. Juice the oranges using a juicer.

3. Serve the juice fresh and chilled.

THIS BLANK SPACE IS INTENTIONAL AND HAS BEEN DELIBERATELY INCLUDED TO ENHANCE THE READING EXPERIENCE. PLEASE CONTINUE WITH THE NEXT PAGE.

Chapter 18: Innovative Juicing Trends

As juicing continues to grow in popularity, new trends and advancements emerge. This chapter explores cutting-edge ingredients, innovative recipes, and technological advances in juicing.

Cutting-Edge Ingredients

New Superfoods and Trends

Spirulina: A blue-green algae rich in protein and nutrients. Moringa: Known for its high vitamin and mineral content.

Adaptogens: Herbs like ashwagandha and maca that help the body manage stress☐s Oil: Used for its potential calming and anti-inflammatory effects.

Innovative Juice Recipes

Spirulina Super Greens

1 teaspoon spirulina powder

1 cup spinach

1 cucumber

1 green apples

1/2 lemon (peeled)

Juice the spinach, cucumber, apple, and lemon, then mix in the spirulina powder for a nutrient-packed drink.

Moringa Vitality Boost1 teaspoon moringa powder

1 orange (peeled)

1 carrot

1 apple

1-inch piece of ginger

Instructions:

Juice the orange, carrot, apple, and ginger, then stir in the moringa powder for a powerful energy and health boost.

Technology and Juicing

Modern Juicing Equipment

Cold-Press Juicers: Preserve more nutrients by minimizing heat and oxidation.

Smart Juicers: Equipped with features like recipe suggestions and nutrient tracking.

Portable Juicers: Compact and convenient for on-the-go juicing. Technological Advances in Juicing

App Integration: Apps that connect to your juicer, providing recipes, tracking, and customization.

Advanced Filtration Systems: Ensure smoother, pulp-free juices. Self-Cleaning Features: Make the juicing process more convenient and user-friendly.

Chapter 19: Case Studies and Testimonials

Hearing from others who have incorporated juicing into their lives can be incredibly motivating. This chapter shares success stories, personal journeys, expert opinions, and scientific studies on the benefits of juicing.

Success Stories

Personal Journeys with Juicing

Juicing has transformed the lives of many individuals, including me, Once a dietitian earning a modest income, I discovered the power of juicing and became a well-known figure in my local community for my juicing expertise.

Meredith's(my journey)

I was passionate about nutrition but struggled to make a significant impact in my early career as a dietitian. When I started experimenting with juicing, I noticed dramatic improvements in my health and energy levels. Inspired, I began sharing my juicing recipes and tips with my clients, friends, and family.

Meredith's Testimonial:

"I was earning very little from my dietetics practice, and it was disheartening. Juicing changed everything for me. Not only did I feel more energized and vibrant, but I also saw real, tangible health improvements in myself and others.

Today, I'm proud to be known as the 'Juicing Guru' in my community. Juicing has not only transformed my health but also my career."

Weight Loss Transformations

Through my juicing workshops and community outreach and through the help of God's knowledge bestowed on me , I helped many people achieve their health goals. One of the most remarkable stories is that of my friend, Emily.

Emily's Testimonial:

"After years of struggling with my weight, I decided to give Meredith's juicing program a try. The results were incredible. I lost 40 pounds in eight months, and I felt more energetic than ever. Juicing helped me stay full and provided all the nutrients my body needed. I am forever grateful to Meredith for introducing me to the world of juicing."

Chronic Illness Management

My cousin ,John, had been managing hypertension for years with medication, but he wanted a more natural approach. So I developed specific juice recipes to help manage his condition.

John's Testimonial:

"Living with hypertension was tough, but Meredith's juicing recipes made a huge difference. My blood pressure has stabilized, and I feel healthier overall. The combination of beet, spinach, and apple juices became my daily routine, and the results speak for themselves. Juicing has truly been life-changing."

Health Transformation Testimonials

1. Weight Loss Success:

"After incorporating daily green juices into my routine, I lost 30 pounds over six months. Juicing helped me stay full and energized while providing essential nutrients." □Sarah, Workshop Participant

2. Improved Digestion:

"I struggled with digestive issues for years. After adding fresh juices with ginger and mint to my diet, my symptoms have significantly improved. I can now enjoy meals without discomfort." ▯Mike, Client

Expert Opinions

Nutritionist and Doctor Insights

Nutritionist:

Nutritionists like Meredith emphasize the benefits of specific ingredients and balanced juicing practices. Meredith often highlights the importance of using a variety of fruits and vegetables to ensure a wide range of nutrients.

Dr. Lisa Patel, Nutritionist:

Doctor:

"Juicing can be an excellent way to boost your intake of vitamins and minerals. By incorporating a diverse range of ingredients, you can ensure that your body gets the nutrients it needs to thrive. And Meredith is an example of someone who understands the secrets to healthy living, her wonderful Juicing journey tells the whole story"

Dr. James Miller, MD:

Scientific Studies on Juicing

Antioxidant Benefits:

Research shows the antioxidant properties of various juice ingredients. For example, studies have found that pomegranate juice has significant antioxidant activity, which can help reduce oxidative stress in the body.

Digestive Health:

Studies indicate improved digestion and gut health from regular juice consumption. Juices containing ginger and mint, for instance, have been shown to alleviate symptoms of indigestion and promote gut health.

Immune Support:

Evidence supports the immune-boosting effects of nutrient-rich juices. Ingredients like citrus fruits, which are high in vitamin C, can enhance immune function and help prevent illnesses.

My journey and the experiences of those around me showcase the transformative power of juicing. Whether it's for weight loss, managing chronic illnesses, or simply improving overall health, juicing can be a powerful tool for achieving wellness goals.

Chapter 20: Juicing for Mental Performance

Juicing can enhance mental performance, including focus, concentration, stress management, and anxiety reduction.

This chapter explores ingredients and recipes tailored for cognitive and emotional health.

Ingredients for Focus and Concentration

Focus-Enhancing Ingredients

Blueberries: Rich in antioxidants that improve brain function. Beets: Improve blood flow to the brain, enhancing cognitive performance.

Green Tea: Contains L-theanine and caffeine, which improve focus and alertness. Spinach: High in iron, supporting oxygen transport to the brain.

Concentration-Boosting Juice Recipes

Blueberry Beet Brain Boost

1 cup blueberries

1 beet (peeled and chopped)

1 apple1 handful of spinach

Juice all ingredients together for a drink that enhances cognitive function and focus. Green Tea Citrus Focus

1 cup brewed and cooled green tea

1 orange (peeled)

1/2 lemon (peeled)

1 cucumber

Juice the citrus fruits and cucumber, then mix with the green tea for a refreshing and focus-enhancing drink.

Stress and Anxiety Management

Calming and Soothing Ingredients

Lavender: Known for its calming effects.

Chamomile: Reduces anxiety and promotes relaxation. Bananas: High in tryptophan, which helps improve mood.

Ashwagandha: An adaptogen that helps manage stress.

Stress-Reducing Juice Recipes

Lavender Chamomile Calm

1 chamomile tea bag (brewed and cooled)

1 teaspoon dried lavender (steeped in hot water and cooled)

1 apple

1 banana

Instructions

Blend the banana separately and combine with the juice of the apple and the cooled teas. This soothing juice helps reduce stress and promote relaxation.

Banana Ashwagandha Bliss

1 banana

1 apple

1 teaspoon ashwagandha powder

1 cup almond milk

Instructions:

Blend all ingredients for a creamy and calming drink that helps manage stress and anxiety.

action. Please respect the rights of the creator by citing or linking back to the original work when sharing or referencing it.

Conclusion

Reflecting on Your Juicing Journey

Tracking Progress and Benefits: As you reflect on your juicing journey, take time to track your progress and the benefits you've experienced. Note any improvements in energy levels, digestion, skin health, or overall well-being. Keep a journal to record your favorite recipes, how they make you feel, and any adjustments you've made along the way. Reflecting on these insights can help you fine-tune your juicing habits and tailor them to your specific health goals.

Continuing Your Health Journey: Juicing is not just a temporary fad but a sustainable lifestyle choice that can support your long-term health journey. Continue exploring new ingredients, experimenting with different combinations, and learning about the nutritional benefits of fruits, vegetables, herbs, and spices. As you integrate juicing into your daily routine, consider how it complements other healthy habits such as regular exercise, adequate hydration, and mindful eating. Embrace juicing as part of a holistic approach to wellness, ensuring you nourish your body and mind for years to come.

Additional Resources

Books, Websites, and Apps for Juicing: Expand your juicing knowledge with recommended resources that provide comprehensive guides, recipes, and expert tips. Explore books by nutritionists and juicing enthusiasts that delve into the science behind juicing, recipe variations, and health benefits. Visit reputable websites dedicated to juicing, offering recipe databases, juicer reviews, and community forums for sharing experiences. Utilize juicing apps that provide recipe ideas, nutritional information, and tracking tools to support your juicing journey wherever you go.

Appendices

Nutritional Information of Common Juice Ingredients

Gain a deeper understanding of the nutritional profiles of common juice ingredients with this comprehensive guide. Learn about the vitamins, minerals, antioxidants, and health benefits associated with fruits, vegetables, herbs, and spices used in juicing. Use this information to make informed choices when selecting ingredients for your juices and to optimize your nutrient intake.

Glossary of Juicing Terms

Navigate the world of juicing with ease using this glossary that defines key terms and concepts related to juicing. From juicer types and techniques to ingredient terminology and health terms, this resource provides clarity and enhances your juicing knowledge.

Index of Recipes

Easily find your favorite juicing recipes with this index organized by category and flavor profiles. Whether you're looking for fruit juices, vegetable blends, herbal concoctions, or spiced elixirs, this index ensures quick access to a variety of delicious and nutritious juice recipes.

References and Further Reading

Explore recommended references and further reading materials to deepen your understanding of juicing practices, nutritional science, and holistic health. This section includes scholarly articles, books, and credible sources that provide additional insights into the benefits of juicing, recipe development, and sustainable wellness practices. By reflecting on your juicing journey, exploring additional resources, and utilizing the appendices provided, you can enhance your knowledge, refine your juicing practices, and continue to reap the health benefits of fresh, nutrient-rich juices. Juicing is more than just a dietary choice☐it's a lifestyle that promotes vitality, well-being, and a deeper connection to your health.

Meredith Anne Greene, MD, began her career as a dietician, passionate about nutrition and wellness but faced challenges with financial stability. It wasn't until she embarked on her journey into juicing that her career truly flourished. Recognizing the growing demand for healthy alternatives, Meredith founded a local juicing store in her community, specializing in nutritious juices and wholesome popsicles for children.

Her store quickly gained popularity, becoming a cornerstone for health-conscious families seeking delicious and beneficial treats. Meredith's entrepreneurial spirit and deep understanding of nutrition enabled her to thrive as both a juicing store owner and a distributor of quality juices. This dual role not only fulfilled her professional aspirations but also provided a sustainable income that transformed her initial struggles into success.

Beyond her literary contributions, Meredith remains a devoted mother, balancing her entrepreneurial pursuits with a commitment to family life. Known for her advocacy of privacy, Meredith believes in the power of knowledge standing alone, separate from personal acclaim. Her humility and dedication to enhancing health outcomes underscore her mission to empower others through accessible and practical health advice. Her journey exemplifies resilience and the profound impact of pursuing one's passion while positively influencing the community she serves.